The Nongovernmental Sector in Disaster Resilience

Conference Recommendations for a Policy Agenda

Joie Acosta, Anita Chandra, Sally Sleeper, Benjamin Springgate

Sponsored by The Allstate Foundation

RAND GULF STATES POLICY INSTITUTE

These proceedings were sponsored by The Allstate Foundation and were developed in collaboration with the RAND Gulf States Policy Institute, and within RAND Infrastructure, Safety, and Environment and RAND Health.

Library of Congress Control Number: 2011923866

ISBN: 978-0-8330-5215-5

Published 2011 by the RAND Corporation
1776 Main Street, P.O. Box 2138, Santa Monica, CA 90407-2138
1200 South Hayes Street, Arlington, VA 22202-5050
4570 Fifth Avenue, Suite 600, Pittsburgh, PA 15213-2665
RAND URL: http://www.rand.org/
To order RAND documents or to obtain additional information, contact
Distribution Services: Telephone: (310) 451-7002;
Fax: (310) 451-6915; Email: order@rand.org

Preface

Lessons from the management of recent disasters underscore challenges that confront federal, state, and local entities in coordinating with and leveraging the strengths of nongovernmental organizations (NGOs) in disaster recovery. A national policy agenda is needed to crystallize the priorities for partnership, coordination, service capacity, information systems, and funding of NGOs in disaster plans for all types of natural and man-made disasters.

On the fifth anniversary of Hurricane Katrina, the RAND Gulf States Policy Institute, in partnership with the Louisiana Association of Nonprofit Organizations (LANO) and with sponsorship from The Allstate Foundation, invited Louisiana's leaders to discuss the role that nonprofits and other NGOs play in disaster recovery, including ongoing community-redevelopment efforts, and in strengthening communities prior to disasters. The goal of the conference sessions was to formulate an action plan of policy and program recommendations that support the active involvement of NGOs.

This report describes conference concepts for federal, state, and local policymakers involved in developing emergency response and recovery policy, as well as national and local leaders of NGOs interested in the lessons learned summarized in this report. The report summarizes the recommendations provided by panelists and conference attendees, with the goal of developing a national policy agenda for NGO engagement. The recommendations presented in this report reflect the comments and perspectives of conference participants and were not developed by RAND. This work was carried out in collaboration with the RAND Gulf States Policy Institute, and within the divisions of RAND Infrastructure, Safety, and Environment and RAND Health.

The RAND Gulf States Policy Institute

RAND created the Gulf States Policy Institute in 2005 to support hurricane recovery and long-term economic development in Louisiana, Mississippi, and Alabama. Today, RAND Gulf States provides objective analysis to federal, state, and local leaders in support of evidence-based policymaking and the well-being of individuals throughout the Gulf Coast region. With offices in New Orleans, Louisiana, and Jackson, Mississippi, RAND Gulf States is dedicated to answering the region's toughest questions related to a wide range of issues that include coastal protection and restoration, health care, and workforce development. More information about RAND Gulf States can be found at http://www.rand.org/gulf-states/.

RAND Infrastructure, Safety, and Environment

This research was conducted within RAND Infrastructure, Safety, and Environment (ISE). The mission of RAND Infrastructure, Safety, and Environment is to improve the development, operation, use, and protection of society's essential physical assets and natural resources and to enhance the related social assets of safety and security of individuals in transit and in their workplaces and communities. For more information about RAND ISE, please visit http://www.rand.org/ise.html.

RAND Health

This work was also carried out within the RAND Public Health Systems and Preparedness Initiative within RAND Health. A profile of the initiative, abstracts of its publications, and ordering information can be found at http://www.rand.org/health/centers/public-health-systems-and-preparedness.html. RAND Health is a division of the RAND Corporation.

Comments or inquiries should be sent to the principal investigator, Sally Sleeper (Sally_Sleeper@rand.org). The mailing address is RAND Gulf States Policy Institute, 650 Poydras Street, Suite 1400, New Orleans, LA 70130.

Abstract

Nongovernmental organizations (NGOs) are instrumental in communities' resilience to natural and man-made disasters. But, despite national progress, the plans and processes for their involvement are not well-defined. This report summarizes three interrelated conference sessions that RAND researchers convened during the Louisiana Association of Nonprofit Organizations annual conference in August 2010. The purpose of the three sessions was to generate a national policy agenda that summarizes the challenges to involving NGOs in disaster response and recovery and to identify potential policy and program recommendations to address these challenges, with a specific emphasis on two types of populations, which were most in need after recent disasters: displaced and returning individuals and individuals with mental health needs. Panelists and conference attendees were asked to identify recommendations that would assist NGO involvement in disaster response and recovery. Those recommendations were then summarized by RAND researchers and were categorized into five areas: defining and formalizing roles for NGOs, structure and integration of governmental and nongovernmental organizations in common plans, information sharing, service capacity, and resource allocation. Based on the conference discussion, this report also contains RAND recommendations for future research to inform implementation of the policy agenda.

Contents

Acknowledgments

We are indebted to the many individuals who participated in this conference and provided their time, expertise, and insights across a wide range of topics related to improving NGO effectiveness and involvement in the process of human recovery postdisaster. Presenters and participants were an informed set of policymakers, practitioners, and academics dedicated to learning from past disasters and applying these lessons to speed human recovery regardless of the nature or location of a disaster. Any errors of interpretation of these participants are, of course, ours.

We wish to thank The Allstate Foundation for sponsoring the conference and these proceedings. Special thanks go to executive director Jan Epstein for her tireless energy and humor throughout the process of shaping the conference. We also thank Victoria Shire Dinges, assistant vice president for public social responsibility at Allstate Insurance Company, for her participation and support.

We are especially grateful to LANO president and chief executive officer Ann Silverberg Williamson and her devoted staff for allowing us to partner with LANO to provide a research-focused conference track during its annual conference.

Several RAND colleagues participated in the conference and we thank them: Mark VanLandingham and Michael Rendall for their research presentations, Kenneth Wells for contributing to the framing of conference session 3 (mental health services and psychological recovery) and the associated chapter, Stacy Fitzsimmons and Lauren Andrews for conference support, and Stacy, in particular, for her careful eyes during the writing of these conference proceedings. We also thank Lisa Sodders and Shelley Wiseman for their contributions to ensuring timely and effective media and presentation materials.

We greatly appreciate the comments from our reviewers, Malcolm Williams and Agnes Schaefer of the RAND Corporation. Their insights greatly improved our report.

Abbreviations

DHS	U.S. Department of Homeland Security
DNORPS	Displaced New Orleans Residents Pilot Survey
DNORS	Displaced New Orleans Residents Survey
FEMA	Federal Emergency Management Agency
HHS	U.S. Department of Health and Human Services
ISE	Infrastructure, Safety, and Environment
LANO	Louisiana Association of Nonprofit Organizations
NGO	nongovernmental organization
NSP2	New Orleans Neighborhood Stabilization Phase 2
PAHPA	Pandemic and All-Hazards Preparedness Act
SAMHSA	Substance Abuse and Mental Health Services Administration
VISTA	Volunteers in Service to America
VOAD	Voluntary Organizations Active in Disaster

CHAPTER ONE

Introduction

As many communities continue to confront stressors from the current economic downturn to the devastation created from man-made (e.g., Deepwater Horizon oil spill) and natural (e.g., hurricanes, floods) disasters, it is critical to consider how these communities develop the capacities and capabilities to respond and effectively recover from such crises. In the wake of these stressors, both government and nongovernmental organizations (NGOs, including nonprofit and for-profit organizations) must be engaged in long-term recovery and community resilience-building activities to improve communities' ability to withstand future stressors. NGOs are the "go-to" entities in disaster response and recovery because of their real or perceived insight on the assets, needs, and sociocultural complexities of their neighborhoods; ability to leverage resources with less administrative hassle for more-efficient response; often-unique access to distribution and dissemination channels for disaster-related information and resources; and ability to support sustainable long-term recovery efforts given ongoing and integrated local presence.

On the fifth anniversary of Hurricane Katrina, the RAND Gulf States Policy Institute, in partnership with the Louisiana Association of Nonprofit Organizations (LANO) and with sponsorship from The Allstate Foundation, invited Louisiana's leaders to discuss the crucial role that nonprofits and other NGOs play in disaster response and recovery, including ongoing community-redevelopment efforts, and in strengthening communities prior to disasters. Over the course of two days, RAND presented key research findings in each of three interrelated sessions and led an expert panel discussion and round-table forum to consider how research can be translated into benefits for the region. The goal of the conference sessions was to formulate a national action plan of policy and program recommendations that support the active involvement of NGOs in all types of emergencies or disasters, both natural and man-made. The conference was organized to elicit concrete and actionable recommendations from panelists and attendees who represented the NGO community and whose voice is often not included in national dialogue.

This document highlights challenges and recommendations that were identified during the conference sessions by panelists and conference attendees, which form the basis of a national policy agenda for improving NGO engagement in disaster response and recovery. The recommendations presented in this report reflect the comments and perspectives of conference participants and were not developed by RAND. The report also provides recommendations from the RAND team for a research agenda that would inform and evaluate implementation of this policy agenda.

Methods

In order to address issues on the roles and responsibilities of NGOs before, during, and after a disaster, RAND convened three conference sessions to summarize lessons learned by NGOs from prior disasters, through the cycle of emergency response into the lengthy long-term recovery process. The goal of the conference was to formulate an action plan of policy and program recommendations to further promote NGOs' active involvement, with specific attention to engagement in the long-term recovery period and to two populations that are critically affected by disaster: displaced and returned individuals, and individuals with mental health conditions. These populations were selected for two reasons. Based on research since Hurricane Katrina (Kessler et al., 2008; Sastry, 2007), we know that individuals are at great risk for displacement and mental health issues as a result of disaster exposure. Second, from ongoing conversations with NGOs (Chandra and Acosta, 2009; Chandra, Acosta, Stern, et al., 2011), we know that NGOs are often on the front lines in locating displaced populations and addressing the long-term mental health needs in a community.

Given this background, the conference sessions focused, respectively, on the role of NGOs in (1) disaster response and recovery more generally, (2) displaced and returned populations, and (3) postdisaster mental health services and psychological recovery. The RAND research team identified three to five members for an expert panel (see the appendix) during each session who would lead a discussion with attendees about issues related to NGO involvement in disaster response and recovery, including, but not limited to, coordination, communication, and financing. The panelists represented federal, state, and local governments, community- and faith-based organizations, and private business. Each session also had a group of approximately 40–60 attendees. These attendees included representatives from all types of NGOs, such as volunteer, faith-based, social services, and disaster-relief organizations; schools; national NGOs; and other community organizations. The attendees also included employers or other for-profit business, but we were unable to include representatives from this business community on each of the three expert panels. The panel for session 2 (displaced population) did include a representative from the housing-finance industry. We acknowledge that future efforts should involve this part of the NGO community more readily, given that these organizations are integral to long-term recovery.

During the panel discussion, RAND and the expert panelists started the discussion by summarizing key themes, issues, and gap areas related to coordination, communication, and financing. Specifically, panelists addressed these questions related to NGO involvement:

- What are some examples of how this challenge (e.g., displaced populations, mental health issues of community members) has affected NGOs?
- What is your vision for what NGO involvement in response and recovery would look like if the challenge did not exist?
- What are the critical policy and program recommendations that would address the challenge?

After each session panel, RAND led a round-table forum to generate discussion among conference-session attendees in the three topic areas. Attendees engaged in discussion in a round-table format. Each round table was assigned a challenge area as a subset of the larger session topic (e.g., for the mental health session, tables discussed prevention, treatment, service coordination) to further address the questions listed above. The goal of the discussion was to generate a list of policy and program recommendations. After individual table discussions, attendees were led in a moderated discussion about the recommendations outlined at each table.

Organization of the Report

The issues that were explored within each conference session varied widely, but it was apparent that NGOs face similar challenges in coordinating and communicating with each other; with federal, state, and local governments; and with other institutions. They share the challenge of working with constrained resources and funding to deliver services and to increase their capacity, staffing, and training. In the next chapter, we provide a synthesis of the key recommendations that emerged from the collective sessions. The policy and program recommendations offered by panelists and conference attendees presented in this chapter are intended to shape the national policy agenda for the effective and efficient engagement of NGOs in disaster response and recovery and in building community resilience to disaster regardless of the type of disaster or the focus of any one NGO. The three succeeding chapters represent each of the three sessions focusing, respectively, on the role of NGOs in (1) disaster response and recovery, (2) displaced and returned populations, and (3) postdisaster mental health services and psychological recovery. Although common themes emerged, each session benefited from the unique insights of its panel of experts and the ideas generated during the round-table part of the sessions. Accordingly, we preserve these with a brief summary of each session. Note that the RAND team provides rationale and further description of each recommendation where appropriate, but these recommendations have not been vetted for effectiveness or reviewed for implementation issues. In addition, where relevant, we have included quotes from conference participants that enhance or exemplify the theme or recommendation. Chapter Six presents areas for research to distinguish which new or different policies and programs are needed to effectively engage NGOs and support the translation of the policy recommendations. These research areas are suggested by the RAND team. The final chapter provides concluding remarks and next steps toward improving NGO engagement in disaster response and recovery. A bibliography of relevant work, including much produced by RAND staff, is included at the end of the document for readers interested in getting more information on these topics.

CHAPTER TWO

A National Policy Agenda to Improve Nongovernmental Organizations' Involvement in Disaster Response and Recovery

The conference discourse illuminated key elements for a policy agenda that should shape the current national dialogue on how NGO engagement could be enhanced or leveraged more effectively in disaster response and recovery. The conference afforded a unique opportunity to consider the policy and program issues confronting NGOs in a structured discussion format that purposefully elicited existing gaps and burdens on NGO engagement. By identifying the gaps, the conference was able to inform a more-strategic vision for how federal, state, and local leaders should discuss NGO involvement moving forward by distilling the key components of that discussion that require the attention of federal, state, and local policymakers. Based on panelist and conference attendee reflections, there are six components:

- Clearly delineate roles and responsibilities for NGOs during each phase of disaster.
- Examine how NGOs leverage routine practice for disaster planning, and identify where opportunities exist for dual benefit in emergency preparedness and daily operations.
- Improve information exchange among NGOs and between NGOs, governmental agencies, and community residents.
- Increase community capacity to deliver seamless, evidence-based services before, during, and after a disaster through NGO partnerships.
- Create guidance about how to allocate resources for NGOs (both financial and nonfinancial).
- Pursue a research agenda that focuses on the implementation of these policy changes and the evaluation of the costs and benefits of NGO engagement.

We briefly summarize these core components here. It should be noted that these components inform an NGO policy agenda not only for disasters but for more-effective engagement of NGOs in strengthening ongoing community resilience. There are many definitions of *community resilience* that center on a community's ability to rebound. In the area of national health security, community resilience entails the community's ongoing and developing capacity to account for its vulnerabilities and develop capabilities that aid that community in preventing, withstanding, and mitigating the stress of an event; recovering in a way that restores a community to a state of self-sufficiency; and allows that community to use knowledge from a past response to strengthen the community's ability to withstand the next event (Norris, 2008; U.S. Department of Health and Human Services, 2009; Chandra, Acosta, Stern, et al., 2011). The recommendations presented in this report reflect the comments and perspectives of conference participants and were not developed by RAND.

Clearly Delineate Roles and Responsibilities for NGOs During Each Phase of a Disaster

Throughout the three conference sessions, the question of how NGOs are reflected in existing national and state disaster policies and guidance consistently emerged. Despite national progress on this front, there are still limitations in the clear delineation of NGO roles and responsibilities in each phase of disaster preparedness, response, and recovery. Further, the expectations, processes, and accountability structures to formally involve particular NGOs in specific aspects of recovery remain elusive.

Examine How NGOs Leverage Routine Practice for Disaster Planning, and Identify Where Opportunities Exist for Dual Benefit in Emergency Preparedness and Daily Operations

In addition to how well NGOs are represented in government plans, there is also concern about how NGOs organize around disaster responsibilities while maintaining routine operations. NGOs are often resource challenged; thus, a policy agenda should examine how NGOs ramp up in response to comparatively infrequent disasters and how this relative balance affects overall organization planning. Plus, NGOs might need to have plans and algorithms that guide decisions about when and how they leverage their partnerships with each other to account for limited resources, organization skills, and capacities, yet for dual benefit. To date, there has been limited guidance or tools to assist NGOs in this type of strategic planning.

Improve Information Exchange Among NGOs and Between NGOs, Governmental Agencies, and Community Residents

Understanding the capacities and capabilities of NGOs and the needs of populations during and after disaster rests on the ability to exchange information seamlessly among stakeholders. The conference highlighted gaps in current information systems. First, the data on population in- and out-migration, displacement, and the needs of those populations are not well linked to organizations providing services. Without that information, NGOs cannot appropriately plan for and respond to changing community needs, particularly in the domains of economic, social, and health recovery. Second, data systems that track the receipt of health and social services are not always matched, despite the fact that individuals often need both sets of services. More-robust data systems that exchange information between behavioral health and social service providers, for example, could reduce service redundancy, verify that individuals are receiving appropriate services, and be used to map service delivery to service outcomes at the individual, family and household, and neighborhood levels.

Increase Community Capacity to Deliver Seamless, Evidence-Based Services Before, During, and After a Disaster Through NGO Partnerships

The policy agenda on the role of NGOs must consider multiple elements of service capacity, including recovery service type and quality, NGO ability to provide services, and evaluation of the delivery of those services. In developing and strengthening a national human recovery system, we must consider what services should be required elements in disaster-recovery planning. This includes service mix for medical, behavioral health, employment, and other social services and must include a discussion of what services are considered culturally appropriate and evidence informed. NGOs' ability to provide services must be assessed in advance of disasters as part of routine preparedness activities, with attention to determining the necessary standards for NGOs to provide certain types of services. This evaluation or assessment has implications for resource allocation but could also inform the type of partnership network described in the previous core component of the policy agenda.

Create Guidance About How to Allocate Resources for NGOs (Both Financial and Nonfinancial)

Another component of the policy agenda must be a discussion of how resources are allocated, the decision rules that guide these allocations, and how these rules remain nimble to a changing context, including disaster type and the nature of overlapping disasters. As such, resources for NGOs (both financial and nonfinancial) should be explored with attention to the maximum level needed by the extent of the disaster and by the type of NGO in receipt of the resources; processes for reducing encumbrances on funding; and accountability for the resources. In addition, consideration is needed about how the for-profit and nonprofit communities can work collaboratively on leveraging and maximizing resources.

Pursue a Research Agenda That Focuses on the Implementation of These Policy Changes and the Evaluation of the Costs and Benefits of NGO Engagement

Pursuit of the aforementioned five policy areas must be accompanied by a robust research plan that monitors and evaluates the implementation of these policies. Outcomes could include improvements in NGO–government coordination, development of doctrine or policies for when and how NGOs are engaged in different phases of disaster, and evidence that funding is used appropriately and effectively. Further, a benefit assessment that provides some valuation on the relative contribution of NGO involvement in specific types of disaster-response and recovery activities would bolster the integration of NGOs in both national and global disaster plans and frameworks.

These six components were distilled from more in-depth discussions that occurred during the three sessions: the role of NGOs in (1) disaster response and recovery, (2) serving displaced and returned populations, and (3) providing postdisaster mental health services and psychological recovery. These discussions focused on the key challenges that NGOs face initiating and maintaining involvement in disaster response and recovery generally (Chapter Three: Session 1 Summary) and when serving vulnerable populations, such as those that have been displaced by disaster (Chapter Four: Session 2 Summary) and those needing postdisaster mental health services (Chapter Five: Session 3 Summary). Recommendations for specific policies and programs—developed during each session—with attention to the first five components are included in the next three chapters. Chapter Six includes research recommendations that, based on conference discussions, were identified by the RAND team.

CHAPTER THREE

Session 1 Summary: The Role of NGOs in Disaster Response and Recovery

Recent national strategies and guidance are increasingly recognizing the roles and responsibilities of NGOs in disaster response and recovery, particularly as there is greater momentum toward formal engagement of NGOs as the cornerstone of building community resilience. Community resilience, or a community's sustained ability to withstand and recover from adversity (e.g., economic stress, influenza pandemic, man-made or natural disaster) has become a key policy issue, especially in the past couple of years (U.S. Department of Health and Human Services, 2009; U.S. Department of Health and Human Services, 2010; National Security Strategy, 2010; Federal Emergency Management Agency [FEMA], 2010; FEMA's Disaster Case Management Program). Although there has always been recognition of NGOs' integral role in bolstering community resilience, as evidenced in the response to Hurricane Katrina, the Haiti earthquake, and the *Deepwater Horizon* oil spill, there is far more emphasis now on understanding, defining, and strategically engaging NGOs in the disaster-recovery continuum or process.

We know from prior disasters that NGOs provide information and referral during and after disaster; are instrumental in providing direct services, including health and employment programs; and often serve as the government link in connecting community members to financial services (Homeland Security Institute, 2006). However, there are two contextual factors that must be considered as NGO roles and responsibilities are more-formally integrated into this national doctrine. First, all disasters are not created the same in terms of the risks that each hazard presents to the community and the needs of the community in response and recovery. Communities contend with a range of man-made (including technological) and natural disasters that can occur at the same time and necessitate different resources and different expectations for recovery. Second, disaster-recovery periods are not discrete and typically overlap. The community and, consequently, the NGOs can be drained of economic and other resources to effectively respond and support their constituents. On the other hand, these NGOs can have enhanced knowledge after a disaster that affords them greater capability to shorten the recovery period of the next disaster because they can more-quickly map community assets and deficits.[1] Addressing these contextual factors assumes that NGOs have relatively unencumbered processes to access local, state, and national resources (both financial and nonfinancial); have the organizational capacity and capabilities to participate successfully in disaster recovery; and have the network visibility to collaborate with other NGOs for the greatest positive impact, with limited redundancy. Yet, these are precisely the gap areas that NGOs identify as being particular impediments to their engagement in long-term recovery (Chandra and

---

[1] See Chandra and Acosta, 2009, for more detail on these challenges.

Acosta, 2009). The session described in the next section sought to understand these challenges and to identify recommendations to address the gaps.

Challenges and Recommendations

Overall, the session yielded a productive discussion that propelled the development of a human recovery system, or a system that supports the return of healthy daily social functioning in a community affected by disaster. The discussion was purposely designed to identify the major types of challenges that NGOs face in disaster response and recovery, while later sessions were focused on specific subpopulations. This session generated two types of recommendations: (1) recommendations that have been voiced before in the ongoing dialogue about Hurricane Katrina and the *Deepwater Horizon* oil spill yet still have not been sufficiently implemented and (2) recommendations in new areas that we need to consider for promoting all-hazards response and recovery capabilities for NGOs. In particular, recommendations clustered into the following areas:

- NGO–Government Coordination and Response Reliability: ways to enhance NGO–government coordination in recovery and identifying which NGOs are best equipped to provide response and recovery services in this system, particularly with respect to behavioral health and social services
- NGO Networks: how NGOs should communicate and partner with each other
- Financing: where financing can be streamlined and improved for human recovery services, and how to develop sustainable funding streams for long-term human recovery, including engaging the foundation and corporate philanthropic communities.

In the next sections, we summarize the key challenges and recommendations provided by conference participants in these three areas.

Area 1: NGO–Government Coordination and Response Reliability

The conference discussion identified several challenges that hampered NGOs' ability to attend to their core roles in disaster response and recovery described earlier. These included difficulties in providing appropriate and comprehensive direct services, such as health and social services. In addition, participants described problems in gauging their responsibility level, particularly with government presence in the early phase of recovery, and in knowing which NGOs were best equipped for specific elements of recovery service provision.

Challenge 1.1: Requirements for Health and Social Services Are Not Well Specified. Despite acknowledgment that disasters often bring unique health and social needs resulting from or being magnified by the stress and trauma associated with disaster exposure, there are still questions about what requirements NGOs should follow to develop their health and social service plan for recovery. Participants acknowledged that they often must cobble together information and guidance from several government sources (e.g., Substance Abuse and Mental Health Services Administration [SAMHSA], Federal Emergency Management Agency [FEMA]) but still lack common, consistent, and comprehensive guidance on the content of health, behavioral, and social services for both the response and recovery periods. Specifically, participants argued that they needed more-detailed plans in the following areas: case management for the long-term recovery period (building on FEMA's Disaster Case Management Program); children's health and social services; behavioral health services for the short- and long-term recovery periods (see session 2); and services to help families reestablish households (e.g., rental deposits, household bills). In addition to lacking the necessary detail for these components of a human recovery system, participants shared that there are still problems in how these services are coordinated via NGO networks and government–NGO partnerships.

Recommendation 1.1.1: Develop a human recovery strategic plan. Although there are now national strategies and frameworks that outline some of the critical elements of recovery,[2] the conference participants contended that there is still a need for a larger strategic plan specifically focused on long-term human recovery that could be embraced by local, state, and federal leaders. This *long-term human recovery strategic plan* would be developed with these leaders, building on lessons learned from past disasters and strategies and approaches that have been deemed successful in terms of community resilience. The strategic plan would outline specific information on who is responsible for key elements of health and social system recovery and when coordination among government and nongovernmental sectors is required. Although there will be community and disaster-type variation in the recovery plans, this strategy would give the necessary frame for human recovery with information on government services and guidelines for "best practice" in health and social service support.

> NGOs need to be at the table from the start, before the start, during the start, right after the start, after the start. We have to be at the table in all of the planning. Whether we ensure that by a statute or regulation in the Stafford Act, we would have to do some research to figure that out.

Recommendation 1.1.2: Develop planning templates and processes for integrating health, behavioral health, and social services. Consistent with the human recovery strategic plan, participants recommended that NGOs would benefit from checklists and templates for concrete guidance on the type of staffing and resources (e.g., curricula, medications, social service programs) needed to integrate health, behavioral health, and social services into their disaster-response and recovery plans. These materials could be used by states and localities to ensure that the right services are planned for and included in the recovery plans, with attention to the resources required (e.g., staff, finances, training).

In addition to templates, participants noted, there should be a better way to link mental health recovery into social service efforts (i.e., a recovery tracking system). NGO representatives shared that having a means of tracking individuals in need of postdisaster social services across agencies to ensure continuity of care and to prevent disconnection from each element of postdisaster recovery services was needed. Although some communities use existing databases (e.g., Coordinated Assistance Network) or their own derived database, these systems still have limitations in what they can track and how agencies use them to develop a comprehensive recovery plan for community members (Acosta, Chandra, and Feeney, 2010). A recovery tracking system could be used as a screening or diagnostic tool that not only documents need but more-consistently maps to existing services. Service availability could be prepopulated before disaster but would also be regularly updated during and after disaster to account for

---

[2] See recovery objective in U.S. Department of Health and Human Services, 2009, and Federal Emergency Management Agency, 2010.

changing timelines of service restoration. The system could also have dual use by providing demographic data for individuals in need of postdisaster services as population levels change with disaster-related in- and out-migration. Finally, in order to support some of this new planning around behavioral health and social services specifically, participants suggested the designation of a local disaster mental (or behavioral health) coordinator.

Recommendation 1.1.3: Continue to modify the Stafford Act and Medicaid to account for emergency health and social service provisions. Participants also called for national policies to further clarify the role of NGOs as part of coordinated governmental response to disasters—in particular, the Stafford Act[3] and Medicaid. The Stafford Act defines when and how major disasters are declared, determines the type of assistance to be provided by the federal government, and establishes cost-sharing agreements among federal, state, and local governments. The type of emergency health and social service provisions currently eligible for reimbursement under the Stafford Act are limited. Although there have been recommended revisions to the Stafford Act, participants shared that the edits did not yet allow for longer-term outpatient treatment of conditions (physical and mental) related to the catastrophic event, nor did the act clearly outline how these services would be funded via preapproved contracts or another comparable mechanism. In addition to the Stafford Act, participants suggested, there should be greater emergency provisions in Medicaid that provide flexibility around eligibility and extend coverage with federal financing in these crises. Medicaid funds medical and some mental health services for low-income families—the same families that are among the most vulnerable to disasters (Donner and Rodríguez, 2008).

Challenge 1.2: Transition points between government and NGOs in recovery service provision are still unclear. Another challenge identified by conference participants was around the lack of specificity regarding the role NGOs should assume during the transition between response and recovery, when federal government support is necessarily waning. More specificity is needed to clarify when in the disaster cycle NGOs should take the lead in delivering which types of services. Despite progress in state and federal policy to more-formally document NGO involvement (U.S. Department of Health and Human Services, 2009; Federal Emergency Management Agency, 2010; FEMA's Disaster Case Management Program), participants shared concerns about lack of detail in the responsibilities that NGOs have, specifically in recovery. There is also very little information outlining a general timetable of when transition points in recovery service delivery should occur and what the metrics are of successful NGO involvement at those benchmark points. In addition, there is minimal detail on transition to recovery planning as part of overall community-preparedness activities and general incident planning.

> Because we all deal in this continuum of care with a broad range of different services and different NGOs and nonprofits providing different services, . . . I may have moved on from response to recovery with this person because [the person is] now receiving assistance in a regular way from one or our regular distribution points as opposed to a special distribution point that's been set up for response.

Recommendation 1.2.1: Develop a formal structure for government and NGO partnership in recovery. In order to address this challenge, the participants suggested, the federal gov-

---

[3]   Robert T. Stafford Disaster Relief and Emergency Assistance Act, Pub. L. 100-707, November 23, 1988.

ernment and NGOs should partner to develop a structure and process for working together. This would include guidelines for integrating recovery planning and capacity building before a disaster to ensure that NGOs have the resources (e.g., financial, staff, training) to execute their roles in recovery. The plan would clarify when government resources would recede and when NGOs should take the lead on service provision so that community-level predisaster plans could adequately account for those transitions in the delivery of recovery services.

In addition to the NGO responsibility and transition-point information, participants argued for a better, single federal model for case management that is clearly defined, responsive to local conditions, accountable, and adequately funded. During the conference session, there was specific discussion about revisions to FEMA's Disaster Case Management Program, and participants underscored the need to ensure that the program is appropriately changed to reflect these elements. Participants also recommended that there be a single federal point of contact for NGO coordination.

Challenge 1.3: Poor identification of "response-reliable" NGOs preincident impedes effective and efficient response and recovery. The session discussion also focused on the circumstances surrounding which NGOs were involved in specific aspects of disaster recovery. Participants indicated that there was a lack of clarity about which NGOs are best positioned to lead recovery service delivery or manage the financing aspects of recovery. Ideally, NGOs would have adequate staffing to handle surge in the event of a major disaster and have done adequate planning to ensure continuity of operations and utilize government funding effectively. An NGO with the broad operational capability to adapt easily in response to changing conditions would be more likely to perform well during a disaster than an NGO that relies on a single supplier or person (Jackson, 2008). There are no standard criteria to determine which NGOs are best positioned for response and recovery. Further, there is no assessment process for determining which NGOs should lead elements of recovery, which NGOs have appropriate surge capacity, and which NGOs have the ability to leverage and track the use of government and other dollars efficiently and effectively.

Recommendation 1.3.1: Develop a process to review the capacity and capability of NGOs, particularly for disaster recovery. As a result of this challenge, an assessment process could be used to specially vet NGOs that want to provide services (e.g., case management). This review would populate a "qualified list" of NGOs so that these organizations can be ready for a disaster quickly and would also inform a set of contingency plans for other NGOs to engage if the primary group of NGOs is overwhelmed due to the disaster. This list could be used to determine predisaster training needs and gaps in NGO capacity, as well as contract for recovery service funding and reimbursement.

Area 2: NGO Networks

Relationships among the nonprofit organizations that are involved in both traditional and nontraditional disaster-response and recovery roles are the second area in which challenges and recommendations cluster. The challenges in this section focus primarily on structure, coordination, and strength of these relationships. Policy and program recommendations in this area offer potential actions to build more-coordinated NGO–NGO partnerships.

Challenge 1.4: NGO–NGO networks are challenged by variation in organizational structure. NGOs vary widely on a number of key characteristics (e.g., the number of staff, staff composition [e.g., professional, administrative, managerial], operating budget, mission and vision) and capacities (e.g., leadership, equipment). NGOs assume varied roles and responsibilities during disaster response and recovery in part because of variations in these key characteristics and capacities (Cutter et al., 2006; Waugh, 2006). During disaster response and recovery, these variations can make it difficult for NGOs to identify shared outcomes and accountability processes. Sharing data between NGOs has been done through such mechanisms as the Coordinated Assistance Network, a centralized web-based database with information about disaster victims and their needs; however, challenges to consistently sharing appropriate and high-quality data still exist (Acosta, Chandra, and Feeney, 2010). Tensions also arise when these NGO–NGO networks try to balance inclusion of all NGOs with agreed-upon standards of conduct that only some NGOs are qualified to meet (see also recommendation 1.3.1). Finally, representatives from NGOs identified the need for guidance and tools to facilitate connections among NGOs and enhance their ability to leverage assets community-wide. The following recommendations are framed as potential actions to address these challenges.

Recommendation 1.4.1: Develop a national database for case management that identifies a core set of shared outcomes. The development of a national database could help prioritize the identification of a core set of shared outcomes and the corresponding measures that could be utilized to monitor and evaluate across disaster case-management programs. As described in area 1, identifying this outcome list for NGOs and recovery generally, and case management specifically, is critical for future research. Implementation of a national database for case management is critical to ensure that consistent high-quality data are collected on disaster victims' needs and services provided. Access to this type of data could help minimize duplication of services and facilitate continuity of care, as well as provide valuable insight into the effectiveness and efficiency of these programs. In order to ensure utilization of a standardized national database, the Stafford Act or National Disaster Case Management Program[4] requirements could be modified to require states to utilize the database. A cost analysis could help determine whether the cost of developing and maintaining such a database outweighs the efficiencies gained as a result of improved service coordination.

Recommendation 1.4.2: Develop guidance and tools to help NGOs better access volunteer service programs. Staff dedicated (at least in part) to identifying appropriate contacts and building relationships with other NGOs are needed to help develop NGOs' capacity for coordination. NGOs have opportunities to acquire additional staff support through volunteer service programs, such as Senior Corps, AmeriCorps, National Civilian Community Corps, and Volunteers in Service to America (VISTA). However, representatives from NGOs identified the need for guidance or tools to help NGOs to better access these programs for the purposes of improving coordination during disaster preparedness, response, and recovery.

Challenge 1.5: Tension exists between response speed and coordination among NGOs. Without a consistent or standardized means of communication, NGOs face difficulties in quickly coordinating distribution of resources without unnecessary duplication—a more-serious challenge during response when resources are often limited. Some models of NGO collaboration are emerging, such as the National Voluntary Organizations Active in Disaster (National VOAD), a member-supported organization that supports the coordination of planning efforts by voluntary organizations responding to disaster. However, current models of

---

[4] Elizabeth A. Zimmerman, assistant administrator, disaster assistance, Federal Emergency Management Agency, Department of Homeland Security, *Disaster Case Management: Developing a Comprehensive National Program Focused on Outcomes*, written statement of testimony before the U.S. Senate Committee on Homeland Security and Governmental Affairs Ad Hoc Subcommittee on Disaster Recovery, December 2, 2009.

NGO collaboration have limited formal organizational structure to support contracting and management of services during disaster response and recovery. To both maximize efficiency of coordination among NGOs and address the aforementioned challenges to coordination, we offer the following recommendations.

Recommendation 1.5.1: Develop an infrastructure to support and deploy volunteers, including a national database that connects all volunteers in crisis and in noncrisis periods. Resources that link interested volunteers with opportunities in their local community are currently available (e.g., the Corporation for National and Community Service's, 2010, website). However, there is not a single nationwide resource where interested volunteers can enter their contact information and get prequalified to serve during a time of disaster (i.e., register). Expanding current resources to include a place where volunteers can register would provide state and local governments access to a volunteer base that could be mobilized both during times of disaster and to complete ongoing community projects during noncrisis periods. Many NGOs already collect information from volunteers with whom they work. State and local governments should engage NGOs to help populate the database and manage volunteers when needed. Working out the details of how volunteers will be managed before they are required to respond to disaster is critical to ensure an efficient and effective response and will be made easier if the number of volunteers and their capacities are known (e.g., can identify where capacities are limited and recruit additional volunteers before a disaster).

Recommendation 1.5.2: Develop a single-point-of-entry system that can coordinate NGO efforts to reduce duplication and improve coordination. A centralized system would improve coordination among NGOs resulting in a more-streamlined and continuous service delivery experience for individuals they serve. This recommendation could build on the qualified list of NGOs described in recommendation 1.3.1. Once this list is developed, it could inform the centralized system. This system could include a national 211, a telephone service currently funded by the United Way to assess service needs and connect families with local providers, and a shared electronic database in which client information could be stored. A system with a single point of entry or intake would ensure that individuals served by NGOs are asked to share sensitive background data only once and could feed into a centralized database in which the information is stored for all future disasters. A centralized system would also allow for a common screening of eligible cases and assignment of clients to tiers based on triage criteria. NGOs might even consider linking this system with data on clients who routinely receive social services. Linking these systems would make it easier to transition clients from disaster services, such as case management, back to routine social services and would provide valuable background information to providers during a disaster (e.g., disaster case managers); however, there could be issues created by federal and state privacy laws that need to explored before a single-point-of-entry system like this can be implemented. A useful model for such a system—the Camellia project—is currently being implemented in Alabama. Camellia uses a shared technology infrastructure that provides a common client view across agencies, supports performance management, connect case managers, and simplifies intake and access to services.

Recommendation 1.5.3: Offer incentives for NGOs to become part of their state or local VOAD. As previously mentioned, VOADs act as coordinating bodies for NGOs during times of disaster. Incentives, such as tax breaks for 501(c)(3)s and discounts on insurance, would help encourage NGOs to get involved with these coordinating bodies in advance of a disaster so that their capacities and capabilities could be fully utilized during an emergency event.

Area 3: Financing

The third area in which challenges and recommendations clustered was around the funding of the recovery services provided by NGOs (e.g., disaster case management). Limited policy and programs in this area and the lack of a clear understanding of the cost of recovery has created a number of challenges for NGOs that we describe in this section. Suggestions for how to develop new financing mechanisms, revise current funding policies, and leverage existing programs are also offered here.

Challenge 1.6: Federal policy does not adequately support financial mechanisms suitable for NGOs. Through NGO experiences in recent disasters, such as Hurricanes Katrina and Rita and the *Deepwater Horizon* oil spill, it has become apparent that the Stafford Act hinders NGO involvement during disaster response (Chandra and Acosta, 2009). There is no existing contract mechanism in place to guarantee NGOs reimbursement for the critical health and social services they provide. Providing services financed through reimbursements rather than up-front funds is often difficult for NGOs that typically do not operate with large amounts of liquid assets. In addition, a study of the disaster case-management program operated by FEMA—the primary federal entity responsible for dispersing disaster-response and recovery funding—found that the financial procedures utilized by FEMA were not flexible enough to account for state variations in financial procedures (Acosta, Chandra, and Feeney, 2010). This makes it difficult for NGOs being reimbursed by the state (with federal dollars) to navigate the duplicative and conflicting reimbursement procedures delaying and sometimes blocking reimbursement for the services they provide. Finally, states affected by multiple disasters face difficulties getting together the required matched funds, leaving NGOs without a reimbursement mechanism. Although the Stafford Act provides a basis for funding NGO involvement during disaster response, at the time of this writing, there was no current federal policy on how to fund NGO involvement during long-term recovery from disaster.

The Disaster Relief and Recovery Development Act (H.R. 3635) was proposed in September 2009 to make needed improvements to the Stafford Act, including requiring the president to "review regulations and policies relating to federal disaster assistance to eliminate regulations that are no longer relevant, to harmonize contradictory regulations, and to simplify and expedite disaster recovery and assistance" (House Report 111-562). Although these revisions are critical to improve the relevance of these policies and programs to NGOs, the bill never became a law. FEMA is currently in the process of revising its disaster case-management program. At the time of this report, no formal revisions had been published. The three recommendations here are meant to supplement and enhance ongoing policy-reform efforts.

Recommendation 1.6.1: Develop an up-front funding mechanism that prequalifies NGOs for reimbursement and clearly outlines covered disaster-response and recovery services and reimbursement rates. As previously mentioned, NGOs need up-front funding available to quickly provide services. Current mechanisms that provide funding to NGOs that must pass through state agencies create delays in the processing and distribution of that funding. In addition, state agencies often take administrative costs out of this funding, requiring NGOs to cover their own administrative costs (Acosta, Chandra, and Feeney, 2010). To address these challenges, an up-front funding mecha-

There have to be severe financing changes to how this money is allocated. There has to be an allowance for up-front money. We can't have cost reimbursements. That's not realistic when we're in a crisis state. There have to be minimal state-agency administration costs.

nism for NGOs should be created to either provide funds directly to NGOs or put a cap on state-agency administration costs. Administrative costs should be included under reimbursable costs for NGOs, particularly during times of crisis and recovery, where usual services might be disrupted necessitating additional coordination. To ensure that up-front funds are distributed to ready NGOs, a prequalification process will need to be established in which ready NGOs are provided, before a disaster occurs, with memoranda of agreement or contracts to deliver disaster-response and recovery services. This funding would link to the NGO-vetting process described in recommendation 1.3.1.

Recommendation 1.6.2: Improve the connection between short- and long-term disaster case-management services and federal block grant funds intended to provide recovery resources. Representatives from Louisiana NGOs indicated that there was frequently a

> The government [needs] to see human recovery as part of [its] job, not just infrastructure recovery. Direct response, case management, and resources for individual assistance [need to] be allowed to be funded under Stafford and the government's understanding of NGO capability and service delivery and the criteria for response and recovery qualifications [need to be] established so that the NGOs can play the role that they are intended to play in the current system.

disconnect between disaster case-management services and ongoing programs for disaster victims. These ongoing programs, paid for by federal block grant funds, offered services and resources needed by individuals enrolled in disaster case management. However, individuals receiving case-management services were not always able to benefit from these programs because case managers were unaware they existed. Establishing a formal relationship between the disaster case-management programs and the social programs funded through federal block grant funds would help more disaster victims access needed services and resources.

Recommendation 1.6.3: Develop a policy mechanism to ensure that local companies and workers are given priority when funds to do rebuilding are distributed. Representatives from NGOs reported that, after Hurricane Katrina, contractors received additional funds to bring in laborers and materials from outside the affected areas. Although some of these materials and workers were needed, participants indicated that there was a large number of local workers that could have been engaged. Policies related to rebuilding need to acknowledge the role of local companies, particularly if it is more cost-effective to engage local materials and workers. An emphasis on utilizing local residents also helps orient rebuilding into a healing, recovery-focused, and capacity-building lens, rather than just a business opportunity. The Gulf Coast Civics Work Act (H.R. 2269) is one example of proposed legislation in this area. This legislation proposed the development of a corporation to employ Gulf Coast–region residents and evacuees in public-works projects to rebuild the region and established job training programs and apprenticeship programs to recruit qualified workers to relocate to the Gulf Coast. Although this legislation did not pass, the need to engage local workers in rebuilding is still an important point to consider in the ongoing policy debate.

Recommendation 1.6.4: Conduct a review of private and public funding to identify additional streams of funding for NGOs. Federal, state, and local funds to aid in disaster response and recovery are constrained by caps and stringent regulations. In order to augment these funds, NGOs need to review the funding landscape to identify additional private and public funding streams that could be utilized to provide needed services during disaster response and recovery. For example, foundations could be engaged to provide funding for research and evaluation to better understand the role of NGOs in the community. Foundations might also be interested in funding staff positions at national disaster-relief nonprofits specifically focused on conducting outreach to local nonprofit organizations to engage them in response and recovery efforts. Insurance providers represent a private industry that could be engaged. For example, the Homeowners' Defense Act (H.R. 3355)[5] proposed to create a revenue pool into which insurers pay. Interest from this revenue pool could then be used to support NGO services during times of disaster response and recovery. Another strategy for generating revenue from the public is to include a check box on tax forms that allows citizens to make a charitable donation toward disaster funds. Much like charitable campaign contributions, these funds would be tax deductible and pooled nationwide.

One final proposed suggestion is that NGOs establish a revenue-generating enterprise utilizing the principles of social innovation and entrepreneurship. These principles, commonly applied in developing nations with less governmental support, follow traditional business practices to organize and launch a business venture with the ultimate goal of improving social conditions. In this context, NGOs would utilize these principles to organize, create, and manage the delivery of disaster-response and recovery services that are financially supported by private businesses and federal, state, and local governments. Research is needed to identify the model of social entrepreneurship that would be most effective for NGOs to deliver disaster-response and recovery services.

Challenge 1.7: Currently, there is no way to estimate response and recovery costs and the proportion of costs that NGOs share. Establishing a formal financing mechanism for NGOs has been difficult, in part, because there is limited information about what are the actual costs associated with disaster response and long-term human recovery. Therefore, calculating what percentage of the total costs should go to support NGO services has been a challenge. Without a clear understanding of the costs, policymakers cannot determine how much to invest in response and recovery efforts and over what length of time dollars should be spent. Although there have been efforts through proposed legislation (e.g., the Disaster Relief and Recovery Development Act, H.R. 3635) to expedite procedures for estimating the costs to repair or replace infrastructure after a major disaster, little attention has been paid to the costs for health and social services needed to promote human recovery.

Recommendation 1.7.1: Establish a national standard to estimate cost of providing response and recovery services. Donations from the public have been an important source of support for direct services. However, there is not currently a national standard that provides guidance on how to establish estimates for the cost of services. Participants reported that this lack of guidance on estimation procedures resulted in inconsistent estimates and threatened the credibility of reimbursements for direct services. Although costs vary across states and within regions, NGOs could benefit from some standardized guidance to utilize when appealing to donors for additional resources to support long-term recovery. To ensure that these appeals are consistent and appropriate, a national standard for estimating costs is needed. This standard could also help inform federal, state, and local governments about the costs associated with health and social services provided by NGOs.

---

[5]   The U.S. House of Representatives passed the bill in 2007. It was reintroduced as the Homeowners' Defense Act of 2010 (H.R. 2555) and placed on the calendar, June 13, 2010.

CHAPTER FOUR

Session 2 Summary: The Role of NGOs in Supporting Displaced and Returned Populations

After Hurricane Katrina, the city of New Orleans and much of the surrounding metropolitan region were completely emptied and evacuated due to the disaster. Five years after the storm, a significant proportion of the people who left the region still have not returned (Sastry, Fussell, and VanLandingham, 2010). In this conference session, the panelists and participants focused on both the challenges of governmental and nongovernmental organizations that *receive* displaced populations, and preparing for and facilitating their *return*.

The panel discussions and recommendations are intended to help guide the elements of the human recovery system (also termed by one participant as the "human services supply chain") to identify, locate, and assist residents in returning to an area and to provide the tools, information, and resources that are needed by the communities that absorb displaced people.

The panelists focused on understanding the reasons for, and trends in, displacement of populations after disaster. The discussions began with findings from RAND's Displaced New Orleans Residents Pilot Survey (DNORPS) (RAND Corporation, 2010a), which was first fielded in the fall of 2006, and the follow-on Displaced New Orleans Residents Survey (DNORS) (RAND Corporation, 2010b), fielded from June 30, 2009, to May 2, 2010. The surveys examine the location, well-being, and plans for the future of people who lived in the city of New Orleans when Hurricane Katrina struck. The group discussed the types of data most needed by NGOs and other entities and how the implementation of the full DNORS (recently completed) will help to fill these needs.

Challenges and Recommendations

Panelists and discussants provided unique insights from Hurricane Katrina on absorbing the displaced and facilitating their return. The diverse perspectives provided by the presenters, coupled with the subsequent round-table discussions, identified a number of challenges and policy and program recommendations to address the challenges, summarized in this section. In particular, recommendations clustered into the following areas:

- Data Systems for Tracking and Location: ways for improving the collection and dissemination of data and information necessary for addressing the needs of displaced and returning populations
- Communication Plans for Displaced Populations: how NGOs can improve communication and coordination with these populations

- Developing Recovery Plans for Displaced Populations: avenues for increasing NGO capacity to respond more effectively after a disaster.

In the next sections, we summarize the key challenges and recommendations provided by conference participants in these three areas.

Area 1: Data Systems for Tracking and Location

Challenge 2.1: Currently, there is no systematic means for obtaining valid and timely information that is required to address the myriad of human recovery needs before, during, or after a disaster. The residents displaced by Hurricane Katrina evacuated with the expectation that they would return to their homes and businesses. As we know, for months after Hurricane Katrina, much of the metropolitan region was uninhabitable. For many residents, months passed before they were able to return and assess the damage for themselves, and others never returned. Grassroots efforts emerged among neighbors, activists, and community groups to locate each other, in part to knit together support groups and mourn the losses, in part to figure out whether and how to return, and in part simply to find out who survived and who did not.

> There is very little information collected longitudinally about how [evacuees] were faring before Katrina as opposed to afterward. . . . We began to think about what types of information would be most useful to planners both in and out of government about the whereabouts and the needs of the people who were affected.

Communities across the country absorbed the evacuees and mobilized their resources in different ways to provide aid. In addition to the losses of property and life, many evacuees lost access to their bank accounts due to damage to local banking systems, access to medications from the absence of electronic prescriptions, and often access to family members because of the lack of records on where people were sent.

Recommendation 2.1.1: Standardize data sets and establish data-sharing agreements among NGOs and, where possible, government agencies. Participants noted that sharing information was the single hardest point to surmount in coordinating efforts between NGOs and with other private and government agencies. Differing formats, data elements, and the lack of sharing agreements beforehand were significant impediments to sharing information that was needed to provide effective and speedy aid to individuals.

Recommendation 2.1.2: Increase the adoption and use of electronic medical records and revise privacy laws during periods of disaster response and recovery. Individuals were dispersed all over the country after Hurricane Katrina. Many lost access permanently to medical histories, medical records, and prescriptions during this stressful time. In addition, participants noted that privacy laws might have kept families apart when hospitals were not able to share information. Public policy that facilitates the adoption of electronic medical recordkeeping would help displaced populations receive appropriate and needed health care from any location. In addition, privacy laws should be examined to identify when and what information can be shared after a disaster with a large number of displaced persons. More research is also needed to understand the potential impacts of amending privacy laws during a disaster.

Recommendation 2.1.3: Develop a central, shared repository of information on the needs of the displaced and returned populations. Human service NGOs and agencies need to know who needs what, and which organizations can provide the goods or services. Even during times of relative calm, organizations have difficulty coordinating information in the human services supply chain. In a neighborhood-based metropolis, such as New Orleans, participants suggested, NGOs should establish neighborhood response centers in advance of disaster. Such a center would collect baseline information before a disaster and follow-up information during disaster-response and recovery phases on the residents in each neighborhood. This information could then be rolled up to higher levels and managed by a central organization. Volunteer staff at the neighborhood response center would receive timely information on available resources and tailored to residents in their neighborhood from the central organization.

Area 2: Communication Plans for Displaced Populations

Challenge 2.2: Communication among governmental organizations and NGOs within the affected region and with other regions housing the displaced population was limited and evolved ad hoc. Communication issues are closely linked with the availability of timely and accurate information on needs and available resources. Whether displaced or returned, communication with residents, with and between NGOs, and with government agencies remained a significant challenge. The city of New Orleans adopted Internet-based council meetings, which continue today, as a means of raising awareness of progress and needs. Representatives from NGOs and government agencies traveled to the major points of population of dispersed residents—for example, in Houston and Baton Rouge—to hold meetings with residents and groups to gather information and communicate about the resources available to returning populations. However, such ad hoc means of gathering information were coupled with ad hoc communication efforts with other NGOs and agencies on the needs identified, resulting in some needs being unmet and others being met in duplicate. The discussions outlined several related recommendations for improving communication with displaced and returned residents and with and among NGOs.

Recommendation 2.2.1: Establish a protocol for communication that is exercised before a disaster and enacted after one. One participant illustrated the evolution of a communication plan with key NGO and government personnel meeting on a regular basis during the disaster to aid in coordination and information sharing.

Recommendation 2.2.2: A communication protocol should appoint a single person in the network to provide the "trusted" message. In Houston, government and NGOs assigned a single person to manage email communication with participating agencies. In addition to sending out information, the receivers of the information understood the information to be official and correct when it came from that source.

Recommendation 2.2.3: Develop a single website to communicate community and human resettlement issues. This is coupled with a single point of contact (group) that communicates with NGOs and other local governments about services available for displaced persons. A central source of information, viewed as a trusted site, helps NGOs and individuals identify and communicate about available resources in a single location.

Recommendation 2.2.4: Develop standard social-networking tools to communicate time-sensitive information. Many people have communication devices, such as cell phones, and the ability to receive text messages. Government agencies and NGOs can help to coordinate efforts by incorporating a plan for using text messaging and other social-networking tools about activities that arise. For example, they could be used to alert groups or individuals of the availability of transportation into or out of a region.

Area 3: Developing Recovery Plans for Displaced Populations

Challenge 2.3: Most NGOs did not have the capacity to meet the human recovery needs of returning populations. Cities that absorbed large numbers of the displaced residents did not have capacity or established processes for managing the influx of needs. Participants observed that the nonprofit organizations that were most effective in meeting the human service needs were those that had a prestorm capacity to manage such demands. Citizen activism spawned in the aftermath of the storm provided much-needed support but, coupled with the arrival and distribution of donations in every form, also resulted in disorganization in the identification of needs and delivery of services. The ability to ramp up existing NGOs to meet needs was a significant challenge identified in the session. As one participant noted, there were not hundreds of social workers in the receiving cities looking for work, so NGOs were tasked with locating and bringing in paraprofessionals and training them to do case management and triage work quickly.

> We knew that we weren't going to shelter people [short term]. We knew we needed a long-term solution for housing . . . to make sure they had stable income [and that] they had connection in their community to social services, churches, mental health services, doctors, schools. . . .

Recommendation 2.3.1: Develop and exercise a local recovery plan for human recovery. Such a plan could includes a self-assessment of NGO capabilities and capacities to deliver recovery services, directions for how NGOs can access public funds for designated recovery services, guidance for how NGOs should interface with state and local government during recovery planning and service delivery, and guidance for how NGOs can work together during the cycle of human recovery.

Recommendation 2.3.2: Develop and exercise a recovery plan on how to increase capacity of essential professions. Participants noted the unmet demand for trained individuals for case management. Participants shared stories of the need for increasing capacity on the ground across a range of activities—for example, for loan processing and refinancing to provide people with time to make decisions about their properties. For-profit and nonprofit organizations were equally challenged by capacity constraints, and participants shared insights on how they met—or failed to meet—such demands after the disaster. The key lesson that emerged was the need to plan for an event, develop training materials and modules, and encourage partnerships with similar organizations in other regions to increase capacity during crisis.

> It's no use having a house if you don't have a school. It's no use having a school and a job if you don't have child care. The comprehensive approach to providing infrastructure is absolutely necessary, including human infrastructure, not just physical infrastructure.

Recommendation 2.3.3: Prequalify NGOs to facilitate funding. The discussions focused on frustrations by NGOs about obtaining needed funding to respond effectively. One solution advocated by participants was to establish a process to certify an organization as capable of performing a particular function. The certification would be used to signal to funders that the NGO is qualified to perform the duties required and reduces the uncertainty faced of resource distributions.

CHAPTER FIVE

Session 3 Summary: The Role of NGOs in Postdisaster Mental Health Services and Psychological Recovery

Of the adults who lived in parishes and counties affected by Hurricanes Katrina and Rita, 49 percent experienced symptoms of psychological distress that could be consistent with actual mental illness using validated mental illness scales (Voelker, 2010). Unlike other disasters, in which mental health symptoms tend to peak at six to 12 months followed by general improvement in reported mental health, there has been an extraordinary persistence of these systems in this population. Children were comparably affected. A recent study of children who have been living in FEMA trailers reports that 40 percent or more of those who lived in FEMA trailers for an extended period of time following the disaster could have longer-term psychological, emotional, or behavioral health consequences with which they are still struggling five years later (Abramson et al., 2010). At the same time, mental health professionals were displaced, clinics were closed, and the workforce was widely dispersed. Surveys documented that there was very limited access to health care and, in particular, mental health care for this population and a significant discontinuation of prior care (Wang, Gruber, et al., 2008).

These facts formed the backdrop for the conference session. The panel and discussion focused on the roles of a wide range of stakeholders (nonprofits; local, state, and federal agencies; researchers; business community; health care providers; faith-based organizations; philanthropy; and others) in developing ways to address the immediate and long-term mental health needs after the disaster, the challenges in attaining capacity to meet needs, and the adoption of evidence-based strategies to improve mental health recovery among disaster-impacted populations. Presentations in part were based on prior RAND research and partnered work on the topics, including an economic model for a comprehensive mental health response to Hurricanes Katrina and Rita (Schoenbaum et al., 2009); community–academic partnerships and other models that can bolster access to high-quality mental health care after disaster (Springgate et al., 2009; Kolko, Hoagwood, and Springgate, 2010; Voelker, 2010); and models for improving quality of mental health care in primary care practices and other common community settings (Wells et al., 2007).

Challenges and Recommendations

Many of the most-significant and widespread population health consequences of disasters and large-scale traumatic events in the United States in recent years arguably have been psychological. Nowhere has this been more evident than along the Gulf Coast, where recurrent hurricanes and the *Deepwater Horizon* oil disaster have battered local communities. To confront this increasingly recognized major public health challenge, new approaches are required of public health officials, policymakers, academia, nonprofits, philanthropy, health care providers, and others, both to mitigate disaster impacts on mental health in the short term and to support psychological recovery for the longer term. Recommendations clustered into three areas, which are summarized here:

- Mental Health Partnerships: how NGOs could partner prior to disaster to increase the infrastructure for responding to mental health needs after a disaster
- Mental Health Workforce: ways in which NGOs can build capacity to rapidly deploy trained mental health workforce in the wake of disaster
- Adoption of Evidence-Based Mental Health Interventions: opportunities for improving the adoption of evidence-based models and practices to increase the effectiveness of postdisaster mental health care.

In the next sections, we summarize the key challenges and recommendations provided by conference participants in these three areas.

Area 1: Mental Health Partnerships

Challenge 3.1: Efforts to mitigate mental health consequences of disaster must include efforts designed to build longer-term infrastructure and capacities for postdisaster mental health services in affected communities. Many communities and states that might be subject to a higher-than-average recurrence of disaster threat (e.g., from hurricanes, terrorism, wildfires, or earthquakes) could be particularly likely to benefit from policies and investments to build longer-term service capacity to facilitate mental health recovery for vulnerable populations. Policy and investment options to support capacities for evidence-based service delivery for vulnerable populations (e.g., previously traumatized groups) could include training programs for regional clinical staff, learning collaboratives for health care providers, and outreach networks involving nonclinical nonprofits and other community-based organizations.

> I think what Katrina and Rita did in many ways was [to lay] bare some of the lax and the deficiencies of our systems [for primary care and mental health care] that were in place pre-Katrina.

Organizational and operational frameworks, such as continuous quality improvement for clinical interventions, could not only offer short-term gains in terms of cost-effectiveness of services and improved outcomes following a disaster but also suggest a framework to guide future responses and means to learn from unexpected or unwanted change.

Recommendation 3.1.1: Improve predisaster partnerships among NGOs that provide mental health services to leverage organizational strengths and capabilities needed to meet mental health demands postdisaster. The shortage of trained health care professionals after the disaster revealed acute gaps in the ability to provide care to those in need. Participants discussed the activities that emerged after the disaster and noted the need to develop strong NGO collaborations and partnerships predisaster that could mobilize postdisaster to meet mental health demands. One example that emerged after Hurricane Katrina offers relevant examples of how predisaster partnerships could be developed (Voelker, 2010). REACH NOLA is a community and academic partnership that was developed in April 2006 with the aim of increasing access to mental health services through partnering with nonprofits, providing funding to nonprofits, and conducting outreach (REACH NOLA, undated). A key to the success of the partnership was engaging the participation of neighborhood faith-based nonprofits, which were a trusted resource for particularly vulnerable populations. The ongoing partnership provides training and outreach to support the diverse partnership and develop human capital for mental health recovery in New Orleans.

Recommendation 3.1.2: Establish partnerships with NGOs that are non–mental health providers to improve coordination of all services and provide wraparound care. Session attendees who had experienced Hurricane Katrina noted that it was difficult for the affected population to manage mental health symptoms, such as depression, amid daily and long-term uncertainty about housing and employment. Models emerged after the disaster to help connect people with health and mental health services and case-management services. The St Bernard Project (undated) evolved from supplying rebuilding recovery and case management to include mental health services to its residents through a partnership with the Louisiana State University Health Sciences Center and is part of the New Orleans Neighborhood Stabilization Phase 2 (NSP2) Consortium—a consortium of 11 nonprofits dedicated to comprehensive redevelopment across the city of New Orleans.

Area 2: Mental Health Workforce

Challenge 3.2: Organizations that typically provide mental health services on a routine basis are not always engaged in disaster-response and recovery planning. Despite federal and state recovery plans that might include a diverse body of stakeholders, many regional and local agencies, NGOs, clinical personnel, and community members are not consistently involved in disaster planning, response, or recovery processes. Trust concerns can be widespread following disaster, particularly among communities affected by historical socioeconomic and health disparities, irrespective of government or other potential recovery partners' intentions. These organizations play critical roles in managing the disaster messages, reducing fear, and ensuring that community members have the support for healthy psychological recovery.

> If people are not depressed and not suffering from [posttraumatic stress disorder], not suffering from anxiety and able to get their businesses going again, able to rebuild their houses more quickly, get their kids back into school more quickly, it's possible that a trajectory of recovery . . . could really be shortened.

Recommendation 3.2.1: Disseminate community-relevant strategies to build capacity and meet unmet needs for population mental health, such as self-advocacy tools for underserved, vulnerable populations (Catalani et al., forthcoming; Chung et al., 2009), and partnered quality improvement efforts to enhance services' effectiveness and organizations' and clinicians' abilities to respond systematically to adverse change (Wells et al., 2007).

Recommendation 3.2.2: Develop training curricula for mental health providers that are tailored to the specific needs of the postdisaster population. Many of the people with mental health issues after the disaster were uninsured and could not access needed care or medications. In addition to trust concerns, overcoming the stigma often attached to seeking mental health care hindered the delivery of services. Clinicians and NGOs realized that they needed different ways to reach the affected population. REACH NOLA, in partnership with others, developed a community health-worker curriculum with emphasis on client engagement. Derived from evidence-based practice, the organization trained about 450 counselors, physicians, and community health workers from about 70 clinical and nonclinical nonprofits.

Recommendation 3.2.3: Establish networks and practices to provide rapid response to fill gaps in the mental health workforce. After Katrina, there was a dearth of trained professionals to supply mental health care needs. Even if care providers had not been displaced, the existing workforce would have been insufficient to meet the demands. Training in place is important for rebuilding capacity. Developing established policy for exchanging professionals in times of crisis was raised as an avenue to explore. Participants also discussed the potential to use telephone-based care to increase behavioral health care capacity quickly. There is a growing body of evidence about the effectiveness of telephone-based care (Wang, Simon, et al., 2007; Hunkeler et al., 2000; Simon et al., 2004).

Area 3: Adoption of Evidence-Based Mental Health Interventions

Challenge 3.3: Evidence-based approaches and other appropriate postdisaster mental health services are frequently underrecognized and underutilized.

> What we have been trying to do [since the storms] is to develop those kinds of services, assertive community-treatment services, attention to case-management services, wrapping around care in terms of care-management services, doing things that are proactive in the sense of picking people up to bring them to their clinical appointments.

Despite epidemiologic evidence of public health and mental health challenges stemming from disasters in the United States over the past decade, public health responses, recovery policies, and recovery programs—whether conducted at the local, regional, state, or national level—often have failed to incorporate or extend the benefits of prior science, knowledge, and experience to improve population mental health outcomes (Kolko, Hoagwood, and Springgate, 2010; Schoenbaum et al., 2009). The following recommendations are expected to improve the impact of the available evidence base and thus the effectiveness of public health approaches to address this national crisis.

Recommendation 3.3.1: Develop targeted educational initiatives on evidence-based mental health practices and services for relevant policymakers, funders, and agency leaders. Such an initiative would convene the relevant parties and researchers on a regular basis to share new knowledge and science, and historical experiences with evidence-supported interventions. It also would be a forum to inform researchers on the needs of policymakers and agency leaders. The convening would provide funding guidance of relevant federal (e.g., U.S. Department of Health and Human Services [HHS], SAMHSA) and state agencies (e.g., disaster-recovery authorities and departments of mental health) and include entities of philanthropic and nonprofit organizations.

Participants noted that significant practical barriers exist for dissemination and uptake of evidence-based practices and services in a postdisaster environment that could be addressed by efforts to improve the awareness of policymakers, funders, and agency leaders. The reasons varied and ranged from a lack of familiarity with evidence-based approaches to a perceived mismatch of evidence-based research to needs in the disaster-impacted environment. The recommended initiative would help to integrate research and evaluation into recovery processes, to identify what models of intervention improve what outcomes, under what conditions, and for which populations.

Recommendation 3.3.2: Forecast mental health services and workforce availability, as well as costs of implementation of models, to improve effective dissemination of appropriate evidence-based mental health care for populations in postdisaster scenarios, and uti-

lize those models to enhance planning and responses for recovery. Service providers and funding agencies often demonstrate complacency and reluctance to invest in systems to learn from their experiences and interventions—whether through rigorous evaluation or research. Turnstile data related to numbers of services delivered are commonly collected, while systems to determine clinical outcome data frequently are deemed too expensive, difficult, or risky to attempt. In addition, there is limited understanding of models of financial support for targeted, appropriate services, and few efforts to integrate existing systems of health care payment into disaster-recovery planning. Models and sources of financial support for mental health services often are planned post hoc, resulting in considerable delay in delivery, and have limited time courses once media attention diverts from the disaster.

Recommendation 3.3.3: Develop community–academic partnerships to conduct community-sensitive, scientifically rigorous, and policy-relevant assessments of unmet mental health need and community priorities. Engaging the research community (e.g., professors from a local university) in the delivery of care provides an additional opportunity to learn from the current disaster and to find sustainable models of mental health care delivery, particularly in vulnerable populations.

CHAPTER SIX

Future Research Opportunities

The conference sessions provided a road map of policy recommendations on how to improve NGO engagement in disaster response and recovery. The discussions also revealed areas in which additional information is needed either to pursue a particular recommendation or to understand more fully the complexity of an issue. For example, several recommendations offer suggested policy revisions that require further research to inform implementation (e.g., what are the specific aspects and implications of amending privacy laws during disaster response and recovery?). Other recommendations require significant investment (e.g., developing a national case-management database) and a cost-benefit analysis would be useful to ensure that the benefits outweigh the costs of implementing the recommendation. In this chapter, we summarize some of the areas for future research that would advance our understanding of the critical role of NGOs in disaster. These areas for future research are not meant to constitute the whole research agenda; however, these ideas could provide a framework for a timely policy-relevant research agenda that could, in part, begin to be studied during the next disaster. Federal agencies (i.e., HHS, U.S. Department of Homeland Security [DHS]) should invest in a comprehensive agenda that delineates research questions that need to be addressed in order to more-actively involve NGOs in disaster response and recovery.

Session 1: Future Research on the Role of NGOs in Disaster Response and Recovery

Areas for future research identified during session 1 cluster into three areas: NGO–government coordination, coordination among NGOs, and financing of disaster-response and recovery services provided by NGOs.

The discussion about NGO–government coordination during disaster response and recovery highlighted several questions requiring more research about appropriate roles and expectations for NGOs before and after disasters. First, research should determine the essential components of health and social service recovery, and those components that are useful but not vital immediately. Second, there is a need to identify a standard set of criteria to determine which NGOs are best positioned to lead response or recovery efforts, to use government dollars effectively, and to handle surge in the event of a major disaster. Building these characteristics into a funding accountability or monitoring system will help ensure that federal, state, and local dollars are invested in NGOs with the greatest likelihood of success. Finally, research that reviews recovery from prior and current disasters should distill the outcomes for successful NGO involvement following disaster. Specifically, research is needed to identify the shared outcomes that signify successful disaster case management and should be tracked nationally. In summary, research questions include the following:

- What are the appropriate elements of a national model of disaster case management, and what are the specific linkages that we should expect between health, behavioral health, and social services?
- What are the characteristics of a response-reliable NGO?
- What are realistic outcomes for NGOs after a disaster, and at what time points, depending on the nature of disaster? What are benchmarks of success?

Improving coordination among NGOs is also a critical task. Research is needed to help identify the key pieces of information needed to prequalify volunteers to fulfill specific roles during a disaster. In addition, studies to examine current models of collaboration and identify the most-effective and efficient structures and strategies could increase NGOs' ability to fulfill crucial roles during disaster response and recovery. The three key research questions that need to be answered to provide the background information needed to improve the process of and systems that support collaboration are as follows:

- What information should be included in the national database of volunteers to ensure that volunteers are prequalified and can be mobilized quickly during times of disaster response and recovery?
- What are the most-effective and efficient models of collaboration among NGOs? How can current models of collaboration (e.g., VOADs) be improved?
- What resources do NGOs need to be partners in these efforts (e.g., what type of technical assistance and training, staff)?

Several questions must still be answered to advance policy and program development related to the financing of disaster-response and recovery services provided by NGOs. First, a comprehensive longitudinal study is needed to identify the costs associated with disaster recovery. A cost analysis should examine not only the services needed but the amount of spending by NGOs needed to realize a given outcome (e.g., moving a family to permanent housing). Once costs are identified the next step is to build an algorithm that can be calibrated according to community risks and damages incurred from disaster to estimate the costs for recovery. Policymakers could use this algorithm when making decisions about how much to invest in preparedness, response, and recovery efforts. This study could also help to identify the critical services that NGOs provide during disaster recovery. Understanding what the costs of these services are could inform the development of a list of covered disaster-response and recovery services and reimbursement rates. Second, research is needed that examines whether it is more efficient for NGOs or for state or local government to lead service delivery during disaster response and recovery. In summary, the unanswered questions necessitating research are as follows:

- What are the long-term costs associated with human recovery from disaster? How much spending by NGOs is needed to realize a given outcome, such as moving a family to permanent housing? How long are federal or state-supported investments in NGO activities needed in the recovery phase to restore communities?

- What are the critical services from NGOs that should be reimbursed by the federal government? What are appropriate reimbursement rates for these services?
- Are NGOs more cost-effective than state or local government in providing services to support long-term recovery?

Session 2: Future Research on the Role of NGOs in Supporting Displaced and Returned Populations

The displacement of residents after Hurricane Katrina posed significant challenges for individuals, on the cities that absorbed the population, and on the NGOs responsible for the many tasks in human recovery. Future research needs identified during session 2 clustered into two key areas: components and guidance for information sharing, and insurers' role in supporting resettlement of displaced and returned populations. There is minimal evidence of the best practices for sharing information about displaced populations. Specifically, there is limited information about what should be shared, how sharing should operate within current privacy laws, and the systems and processes that need to be in place before a disaster to enable information sharing. Furthermore, little is known about the effective incentives for engaging insurers in resettlement of displaced population and models of collaboration between insurers and the federal government. We outline in this section some key areas in which additional research is warranted to improve the recovery of populations who are displaced during a disaster.

- What types of tools and data sets are needed to promote human recovery in the event of large-scale displacements? How can data be shared locally, regionally, and nationally, and who should collect and have access to the tools and information?
- How can evacuation processes be improved to minimize the impact on evacuees, regardless of the length of displacement?
- Under what conditions should privacy laws be eased? What are the potential benefits and drawbacks? Are there other ways to ensure privacy?
- What are the essential pieces of information that NGOs need about the displaced population before an evacuation and subsequent to one?
- How can continuity be improved in the communication between federal agencies and NGOs?
- How can the federal government and private insurers work together more effectively to promote more-expedient resettlement? What would a federal disaster insurance program entail?

Session 3: Future Research on the Role of NGOs in Postdisaster Mental Health Services and Psychological Recovery

Drawing from the lessons learned about how to engage diverse populations in mental health care, discussants agreed that there was still more work to be done to understand the effectiveness of different models for providing postdisaster mental health services and to identify populations with unmet needs. Engaging the research community in the delivery of care provides an additional opportunity to learn from the current disaster and to find sustainable models of mental health care delivery, particularly in vulnerable populations. Research in the following areas would help to support future delivery of postdisaster mental health services:

- What are the best practices and means for transferring evidenced-based research findings related to mental health care into clinical settings?
- How can lessons learned from providing mental health services during disaster recovery be integrated into approaches used during noncrisis periods? When is it appropriate to sustain these models during these noncrisis periods?
- What policies are needed to promote psychological recovery at the population level?
- What incentives or policies will promote the building and retention of networks for mental health care delivery?
- What incentives or policies will promote the building of mental health capacity to respond to crises in any region?
- What are the critical elements that link community-engagement strategies to appropriate mental health care?

CHAPTER SEVEN

Next Steps and Conclusion

Recent national strategies and guidance are increasingly recognizing the roles and responsibilities of NGOs in disaster response and recovery, particularly as there is greater momentum toward formal engagement of NGOs as the cornerstone of building community resilience (U.S. Department of Health and Human Services, 2009, 2010; National Security Strategy, 2010; Federal Emergency Management Agency, 2010; FEMA's Disaster Case Management Program).

This document summarized three conference sessions and, in doing so, has outlined a vital national policy agenda that, if implemented, could ensure that NGOs are effectively involved partners in disaster response and recovery—with particular attention to supporting displaced and returned populations, and addressing population-level mental health needs. Specifically, these conference proceedings have identified five areas that require the attention of federal, state, and local policymakers and leaders:

- Clearly delineate roles and responsibilities for NGOs during each phase of disaster.
- Examine how NGOs leverage routine practice for disaster planning, and identify where opportunities exist for dual benefit in emergency preparedness and daily operations.
- Improve information exchange among NGOs and between NGOs, governmental agencies, and community residents.
- Increase community capacity to deliver seamless, evidence-based services before, during, and after a disaster through NGO partnerships.
- Create guidance about how to allocate resources for NGOs (both financial and nonfinancial).
- Pursue a research agenda that focuses on the implementation of these policy changes and the evaluation of the costs and benefits of NGO engagement.

Many of the recommendations generated will be useful in revisions to the Stafford Act, FEMA's Disaster Case Management Program, Pandemic and All-Hazards Preparedness Act (PAHPA) (Pub. L. 109-417), content of national disaster-recovery plans, and other aspects of human recovery, including the provision of behavioral health and other human health services articulated by HHS, among other agencies. It should also be noted that these components inform an NGO policy agenda not only for a variety of man-made and natural disasters but for more-effective engagement of NGOs in strengthening ongoing community resilience.

The recommendations developed in this document will be shared with national leaders via a congressional briefing. As stated at the outset, these recommendations have not been evaluated for effectiveness, but the research plan presented in Chapter Six could inform this assessment as strategies are tested. Opportunities for future research are detailed in this document and focus primarily on identifying effective models to improve communication among NGOs and between NGOs, governmental agencies, and community residents; collaboration among these same groups; and recovery of vulnerable populations, especially displaced and returned individuals and those with mental health needs. These next steps are critical if the nation is to improve the way in which it enlists and partners with NGOs for strengthening community resilience. Implementing the national policy agenda will provide the intellectual space to answer key evaluation questions about the specific contributions and cost savings potentially conferred by certain types of NGO engagement. In so doing, we will be better equipped to leverage NGOs in ways that will significantly reduce the length and extent of community-level disaster recovery.

Expert Panel Members, by Session

Session 1: The Role of NGOs in Disaster Response and Recovery

Researchers, panelists, and moderators: Anita Chandra and Joie Acosta (RAND), Charmaine Caccioppi (United Way), James Kelly (Catholic Charities), Marsha Meeks Kelly (Mississippi Commission for Volunteer Service), Kay Wilkins (American Red Cross), Mike Manning (Greater Baton Rouge Food Bank), Tom Costanza (Catholic Charities), Zack Rosenburg (St Bernard Project), Gina Warner (Afterschool Partnership), Melissa Flournoy (Louisiana Progress)

Session 2: The Role of NGOs in Supporting Displaced and Returned Populations

Researchers, panelists, and moderators: Mark VanLandingham and Michael Rendall (RAND), Ann Hilbig (Neighborhood Centers, Inc.), Tim Carpenter (Fannie Mae), James Carter (former New Orleans city councilman), Tina Marquardt (Beacon of Hope), Alexandra Priebe (Tulane), Zack Rosenburg (St Bernard Project), Keith Liederman (Kingsley House), Melissa Flournoy (Louisiana Progress)

Session 3: The Role of NGOs in Providing Postdisaster Mental Health Services and Psychological Recovery

Researchers, panelists, and moderators: Ben Springgate (RAND), Daniel Dodgen (HHS), Tony Speier (Louisiana Department of Health and Hospitals), Calvin Johnson (Metropolitan Human Services District), Joseph Kimbrell (Louisiana Public Health Institute), Elmore Rigamer (Catholic Charities of New Orleans), Donisha Dunn (Tulane), Katrina Badger (REACH NOLA), Diana Meyers (St. Anna Medical Mission), Sarah Hoffpauir (LA Public Health Institute)

Bibliography

Abramson, David M., Yoon Soo Park, Tasha Stehling-Ariza, and Irwin Redlener, "Children as Bellwethers of Recovery: Dysfunctional Systems and the Effects of Parents, Households, and Neighborhoods on Serious Emotional Disturbance in Children After Hurricane Katrina," *Disaster Medicine and Public Health Preparedness*, Vol. 4, Supp. 1, 2010, pp. S17–S27.

Acosta, Joie, Anita Chandra, and Kevin Carter Feeney, *Navigating the Road to Recovery: Assessment of the Coordination, Communication, and Financing of the Disaster Case Management Pilot in Louisiana*, Santa Monica, Calif.: RAND Corporation, TR-849-LRA, 2010. As of February 17, 2011:
http://www.rand.org/pubs/technical_reports/TR849.html

Bentham, W., S. D. Vannoy, K. Badger, A. Wennerstrom, and B. Springgate, "Opportunities and Challenges of Implementing Collaborative Mental Health Care in Post-Katrina New Orleans," *Ethnicity and Disease*, forthcoming.

Catalani, C., L. Campbell, S. Herbst, B. Springgate, B. Butler, and M. Minkler, "VideoVoice: Assessing Community Needs and Assets in Post-Katrina New Orleans," *Health Promotion and Practice*, forthcoming.

Chandra, Anita, and Joie Acosta, *The Role of Nongovernmental Organizations in Long-Term Human Recovery After Disaster: Reflections from Louisiana Four Years After Hurricane Katrina*, Santa Monica, Calif.: RAND Corporation, OP-277-RC, 2009. As of February 17, 2011:
http://www.rand.org/pubs/occasional_papers/OP277.html

Chandra, Anita, Joie Acosta, Lisa S. Meredith, Katherine Sanches, Stefanie Stern, Lori Uscher-Pines, Malcolm V. Williams, and Douglas Yeung, *Understanding Community Resilience in the Context of National Health Security: A Literature Review*, Santa Monica, Calif.: RAND Corporation, WR-737-DHHS, February 2010. As of February 17, 2011:
http://www.rand.org/pubs/working_papers/WR737.html

Chandra, Anita, Joie Acosta, Stefanie Stern, Lori Uscher-Pines, Malcolm V. Williams, Douglas Yeung, Jeffrey Garnett, and Lisa S. Meredith, *Building Community Resilience to Disasters: A Way Forward to Enhance National Health Security*, Santa Monica, Calif.: RAND Corporation, TR-915-DHHS, 2011. As of February 21, 2011:
http://www.rand.org/pubs/technical_reports/TR915.html

Chung, B., L. Jones, A. Jones, C. E. Corbett, T. Booker, K. B. Wells, and B. Collins, "Using Community Arts Events to Enhance Collective Efficacy and Community Engagement to Address Depression in an African American Community," *American Journal of Public Health*, Vol. 99, No. 2, February 2009, pp. 237–244.

Corporation for National and Community Service, home page, last updated May 24, 2010. As of February 18, 2011:
http://www.serve.gov/

Cutter, Susan L., Christopher T. Emrich, Jerry T. Mitchell, Bryan J. Boruff, Melanie Gall, Mathew C. Schmidtlein, Christopher G. Burton, and Ginni Melton, "The Long Road Home: Race, Class, and Recovery from Hurricane Katrina," *Environment: Science and Policy for Sustainable Development*, Vol. 48, No. 2, March 2006, pp. 8–20.

Donner, William, and Havidán Rodríguez, "Population Composition, Migration and Inequality: The Influence of Demographic Changes on Disaster Risk and Vulnerability," *Social Forces*, Vol. 87, No. 2, December 2008, pp. 1089–1114.

Federal Emergency Management Agency, *National Disaster Recovery Framework: Draft*, Washington, D.C., FEMA-2010-0004-0001, February 5, 2010. As of January 24, 2011:
http://www.regulations.gov/#!docketDetail;dct=FR+PR+N+O+SR;rpp=10;so=DESC;sb=postedDate;po=0;D=FEMA-2010-0004

Homeland Security Institute, *Heralding Unheard Voices: The Role of Faith-Based Organizations and Nongovernmental Organizations During Disasters—Final Report*, Arlington, Va., December 18, 2006. As of February 17, 2011:
http://www.homelandsecurity.org/hsireports/Herald_Unheard_Voices.pdf

H.R. (House Report) 111-562—*See* U.S. House of Representatives, 2010b.

H.R. 2269—*See* U.S. House of Representatives, 2009a.

H.R. 2555—*See* U.S. House of Representatives, 2010a.

H.R. 3355—*See* U.S. House of Representatives, 2007.

H.R. 3635—*See* U.S. House of Representatives, 2009b.

Hunkeler, Enid M., Joel F. Meresman, William A. Hargreaves, B. Fireman, W. H. Berman, A. J. Kirsch, J. Groebe, S. W. Hurt, P. Braden, M. Getzell, P. A. Feigenbaum, T. Peng, and M. Salzer, "Efficacy of Nurse Telehealth Care and Peer Support in Augmenting Treatment of Depression in Primary Care," *Archives of Family Medicine*, Vol. 9, No. 8, August 2000, pp. 700–708.

Jackson, Brian A., *The Problem of Measuring Emergency Preparedness: The Need for Assessing "Response Reliability" as Part of Homeland Security Planning*, Santa Monica, Calif.: RAND Corporation, OP-234-RC, 2008. As of February 17, 2011:
http://www.rand.org/pubs/occasional_papers/OP234.html

Jones, Loretta, and Kenneth Wells, "Strategies for Academic and Clinician Engagement in Community-Participatory Partnered Research," *Journal of the American Medical Association*, Vol. 297, No. 4, January 24–31, 2007, pp. 407–410.

Kessler, Ronald C., Sandro Galea, Michael J. Gruber, Nancy A. Sampson, Robert J. Ursano, and Simon Wessely, "Trends in Mental Illness and Suicidality After Hurricane Katrina," *Molecular Psychiatry*, Vol. 13, No. 4, April 2008, pp. 374–384.

Kolko, David J., Kimberly Eaton Hoagwood, and Benjamin Springgate, "Treatment Research for Children and Youth Exposed to Traumatic Events: Moving Beyond Efficacy to Amp Up Public Health Impact," *General Hospital Psychiatry*, Vol. 32, No. 5, September–October 2010, pp. 465–476.

Ngo, V. K., A. Centanni, E. Wong, A. Wennerstrom, and J. Miranda, "Building Capacity for Cognitive Behavioral Therapy Delivery in Resource Poor Disaster Impacted Contexts," *Ethnicity and Disease*, forthcoming.

Norris, Fran H., Susan P. Stevens, Betty Pfefferbaum, Karen F. Wyche, and Rose L. Pfefferbaum, "Community Resilience as a Metaphor, Theory, Set of Capacities, and Strategy for Disaster Readiness," *American Journal of Community Psychology*, Vol. 41, No. 1–2, 2008, pp. 127–150.

Obama, Barack, *National Security Strategy*, Washington, D.C.: White House, May 2010. As of February 21, 2011:
http://www.whitehouse.gov/sites/default/files/rss_viewer/national_security_strategy.pdf

Public Law 100-707, Robert T. Stafford Disaster Relief and Emergency Assistance Act, November 23, 1988.

Public Law 109-417, Pandemic and All-Hazards Preparedness Act, December 19, 2006. As of February 18, 2011:
http://thomas.loc.gov/cgi-bin/bdquery/z?d109:S3678:

RAND Corporation, "The Displaced New Orleans Residents Survey: Pilot Study," last modified September 17, 2010a. As of February 18, 2011:
http://www.rand.org/labor/projects/dnors/dnorps.html

———, "The Displaced New Orleans Residents Survey (DNORS)," last modified September 17, 2010b. As of February 18, 2011:
http://www.rand.org/labor/projects/dnors.html

REACH NOLA, "About Us," undated web page. As of February 18, 2011:
http://reachnola.org/about.php

Sastry, Narayan, *Tracing the Effects of Hurricane Katrina on the Population of New Orleans: The Displaced New Orleans Residents Pilot Study*, Santa Monica, Calif.: RAND Corporation, WR-483, April 2007. As of February 17, 2011:
http://www.rand.org/pubs/working_papers/WR483.html

Sastry, Narayan, Elizabeth Fussell, and Mark VanLandingham, *How Fare the Displaced and Returned Residents of New Orleans? Results of an Innovative Pilot Survey*, Santa Monica, Calif.: RAND Corporation, RB-9500, January 2010. As of February 17, 2011:
http://www.rand.org/pubs/research_briefs/RB9500.html

Sastry, Narayan, and Christine E. Peterson, *The Displaced New Orleans Residents Survey Questionnaire*, Santa Monica, Calif.: RAND Corporation, WR-797/2-DNORS, October 2010. As of February 17, 2011:
http://www.rand.org/pubs/working_papers/WR797z2.html

Schoenbaum, Michael, Brittany Butler, Sheryl Kataoka, Grayson Norquist, Benjamin Springgate, Greer Sullivan, Naihua Duan, Ronald C. Kessler, and Kenneth Wells, "Promoting Mental Health Recovery After Hurricanes Katrina and Rita: What Can Be Done at What Cost," *Archives of General Psychiatry*, Vol. 66, No. 8, August 2009, pp. 906–914.

Simon, Gregory E., Evette J. Ludman, Steve Tutty, Belinda Operskalski, and Michael Von Korff, "Telephone Psychotherapy and Telephone Care Management for Primary Care Patients Starting Antidepressant Treatment: A Randomized Controlled Trial," *Journal of the American Medical Association*, Vol. 292, No. 8, August 25, 2004, pp. 935–942.

Springgate, Benjamin F., Charles Allen, Catherine Jones, Shaula Lovera, Diana Meyers, Larry Campbell, Lawrence A. Palinkas, and Kenneth B. Wells, "Rapid Community Participatory Assessment of Health Care in Post-Storm New Orleans," *American Journal of Preventive Medicine*, Vol. 37, No. 6, Supp. 1, November 2009, pp. S237–S243.

St Bernard Project, undated home page. As of February 18, 2011:
http://www.stbernardproject.org/v158/

U.S. Department of Health and Human Services, *National Health Security Strategy of the United States of America*, Washington, D.C., December 2009. As of January 24, 2011:
http://www.phe.gov/Preparedness/planning/authority/nhss/strategy/Documents/nhss-final.pdf

———, *Biennial Implementation Plan for the National Health Security Strategy of the United States of America*, July 19, 2010. As of January 24, 2011:
http://www.phe.gov/Preparedness/planning/authority/nhss/comments/Documents/nhssbip-draft-100719.pdf

U.S. Government Accountability Office, *Disaster Assistance: Greater Coordination and an Evaluation of Programs' Outcomes Could Improve Disaster Case Management—Report to Congressional Requesters*, Washington, D.C., GAO-09-561, July 2009. As of February 21, 2011:
http://purl.access.gpo.gov/GPO/FDLP544

U.S. House of Representatives, Homeowners' Defense Act of 2007, H.R. 3355, 110th Congress, referred to U.S. Senate Committee on Banking, Housing, and Urban Affairs, November 13, 2007. As of February 18, 2011:
http://thomas.loc.gov/cgi-bin/bdquery/z?d110:h3355:

———, Gulf Coast Civic Works Act, H.R. 2269, 111th Congress, referred to U.S. House of Representatives Subcommittee on Workforce Protections, June 11, 2009a. As of February 21, 2011:
http://thomas.loc.gov/cgi-bin/bdquery/z?d111:h2269:

———, Disaster Relief and Recovery Development Act of 2009, H.R. 3635, 111th Congress, referred to Subcommittee on Economic Development, Public Buildings and Emergency Management, September 24, 2009b. As of February 17, 2011:
http://thomas.loc.gov/cgi-bin/bdquery/z?d111:h3635:

———, Homeowners' Defense Act of 2010, H.R. 2555, 111th Congress, placed on the calendar July 13, 2010a. As of February 21, 2011:
http://thomas.loc.gov/cgi-bin/bdquery/z?d111:h2555:

———, *Disaster Response, Recovery, and Mitigation Enhancement Act of 2009*, House Report 111-562, July 22, 2010b. As of February 24, 2011:
http://www.gpo.gov/fdsys/pkg/CRPT-111hrpt562/pdf/CRPT-111hrpt562.pdf

Voelker, Rebecca, "Memories of Katrina Continue to Hinder Mental Health Recovery in New Orleans," *Journal of the American Medical Association*, Vol. 304, No. 8, August 25, 2010, pp. 841–843.

Wang, Philip S., Michael J. Gruber, Richard E. Powers, Michael Schoenbaum, Anthony H. Speier, Kenneth B. Wells, and Ronald C. Kessler, "Disruption of Existing Mental Health Treatments and Failure to Initiate New Treatment After Hurricane Katrina," *American Journal of Psychiatry*, Vol. 165, No. 1, January 2008, pp. 34–41.

Wang, Philip S., Gregory E. Simon, Jerry Avorn, Francisca Azocar, Evette J. Ludman, Joyce McCulloch, Maria Z. Petukhova, and Ronald C. Kessler, "Telephone Screening, Outreach, and Care Management for Depressed Workers and Impact on Clinical and Work Productivity Outcomes: A Randomized Controlled Trial," *Journal of the American Medical Association*, Vol. 298, No. 12, September 26, 2007, pp. 1401–1411.

Waugh, William L., Jr., "The Political Costs of Failure in the Katrina and Rita Disasters," *Annals of the American Society of Political and Social Science*, Vol. 604, No. 1, March 2006, pp. 10–25.

Wells, Kenneth B., Cathy D. Sherbourne, Jeanne Miranda, Lingqi Tang, Bernadette Benjamin, and Naihua Duan, "The Cumulative Effects of Quality Improvement for Depression on Outcome Disparities Over 9 Years: Results from a Randomized, Controlled Group-Level Trial," *Medical Care*, Vol. 45, No. 11, November 2007, pp. 1052–1059.

Wennerstrom, A., S. D. Vannoy, C. Allen, D. Meyers, E. O'Toole, K. Wells, and B. Springgate, "Community-Based Participatory Development of a Community Health Worker Mental Health Outreach Role to Extend Collaborative Care in Post-Katrina New Orleans," *Ethnicity and Disease*, forthcoming.

Yun, Katherine, Nicole Lurie, and Pamela S. Hyde, "Moving Mental Health into the Disaster-Preparedness Spotlight," *New England Journal of Medicine*, Vol. 363, No. 13, September 23, 2010, pp. 1193–1195.

Zimmerman, Elizabeth A., assistant administrator, disaster assistance, Federal Emergency Management Agency, Department of Homeland Security, *Disaster Case Management: Developing a Comprehensive National Program Focused on Outcomes*, written statement of testimony before the U.S. Senate Committee on Homeland Security and Governmental Affairs Ad Hoc Subcommittee on Disaster Recovery, December 2, 2009.